Healthy Eating on a Budget: Nutritious Meals Without Breaking the Bank

By Anthony Colasante

Table of Contents

-

Managing Food Allergies Without Overspending

-

Kid-Friendly Meals on a Budget

Chapter 10: Long-Term Strategies for Eating Healthy on a Budget

-

Building a Sustainable Grocery Budget

-

The Importance of Seasonal and Local Eating

-

Growing Your Own Food at Home

-

Resources and Tools for Continued Success

Conclusion

-

Recap and Final Thoughts

-

Encouragement for Your Budget-Friendly Healthy Eating Journey

-

Additional Resources and Recommended Reading

Appendices

-

Grocery List Templates

-

Meal Planning Templates

Introduction

The Importance of Eating Healthy on a Budget

In today's fast-paced world, it's easy to fall into the trap of believing that eating healthy is expensive or time-consuming. With rising food costs and busy schedules, many people feel that their only option is to choose convenience over nutrition. However, eating healthy doesn't have to mean spending a fortune or hours in the kitchen. In fact, with a bit of planning and smart shopping, it's entirely possible to enjoy nutritious, delicious meals without breaking the bank.

Healthy eating is not just about looking good or staying fit; it's about fueling your body with the nutrients it needs to function at its best. When you eat well, you're not only improving your physical health but also boosting your mental clarity, energy levels, and overall well-being. This book aims to dispel the myth that healthy eating is only for those with deep pockets and to provide you with practical strategies to make it accessible for everyone, regardless of budget.

How to Use This Book

"Healthy Eating on a Budget: Nutritious Meals Without Breaking the Bank" is designed to be your go-to guide for creating affordable, healthy meals. Whether you're new to cooking or a seasoned chef looking to cut costs, this book offers something for everyone. Here's how you can make the most of it:

- **Start with the Basics**: If you're new to budgeting for food or unsure about what constitutes a balanced diet, begin with Chapter 1, where we cover the fundamentals of nutrition and budget-friendly eating.
-

Plan and Shop Smart: Chapters 2 and 3 provide you with the tools you need to plan your meals and grocery shop efficiently. These sections are packed with tips on how to stretch your dollar without sacrificing quality.

-

Dive into Recipes: The heart of this book lies in the recipes. Organized by meal type—from breakfast to desserts—you'll find a variety of dishes that are both healthy and budget-friendly. Feel free to jump to any chapter that suits your immediate needs.

-

Special Considerations: For those with dietary restrictions or specific health goals, Chapter 9 offers tailored advice and recipes to help you maintain your dietary needs without overspending.

-

Long-Term Success: Finally, Chapter 10 focuses on sustainable strategies for maintaining a healthy diet on a budget in the long run. This section is particularly helpful if you're looking to make lasting changes to your eating habits and grocery spending.

Throughout this book, you'll find practical tips, grocery lists, and meal planning templates to assist you in your journey. Each recipe is designed with affordability and nutrition in mind, ensuring that you can eat well without stretching your budget too thin.

The Benefits of Planning and Smart Shopping

One of the key themes of this book is the power of planning and smart shopping. By taking the time to plan your meals and shop with a strategy, you can significantly reduce food waste, avoid unnecessary purchases, and make the most of every dollar you spend.

Meal planning allows you to create a roadmap for your week, ensuring that you have everything you need to prepare healthy meals without the last-minute scramble. It also helps you take advantage of bulk buying, seasonal produce, and sales, all of which contribute to substantial savings over time.

Smart shopping is about making informed choices at the grocery store. This means understanding how to read food labels, knowing which items to buy in bulk, and recognizing when a sale is truly a good deal. It's also about being mindful of your budget and resisting the urge to make impulse purchases that can quickly add up.

By mastering these skills, you'll not only save money but also enjoy a more organized and stress-free approach to eating well. This book is here to guide you through each step, providing you with the knowledge and confidence to make healthy eating on a budget a reality.

Chapter 1: Understanding the Basics of Budget-Friendly Nutrition

The Fundamentals of a Balanced Diet

A balanced diet is the cornerstone of good health, providing your body with the essential nutrients it needs to function optimally. But what exactly does a balanced diet look like, and how can you achieve it without overspending?

At its core, a balanced diet includes a variety of foods from all the major food groups: fruits, vegetables, grains, proteins, and dairy (or dairy alternatives). Each of these groups contributes different nutrients that are vital for maintaining health:

- **Fruits and Vegetables**: These should make up a large portion of your daily intake. They are rich in vitamins, minerals, and fiber, which are crucial for maintaining a healthy digestive system, boosting immunity, and preventing chronic diseases. Aim for a variety of colors on your plate to ensure you're getting a wide range of nutrients.

- **Grains**: Whole grains, such as brown rice, quinoa, oats, and whole wheat, are excellent sources of energy, fiber, and essential nutrients like B vitamins and iron. Choosing whole grains over refined grains helps maintain energy levels and keeps you fuller for longer.

- **Proteins**: Protein is essential for building and repairing tissues, producing enzymes, and supporting immune function. Include a mix of protein sources in your diet, such as lean meats, poultry, fish, eggs, beans, lentils, and nuts. Plant-based proteins can be more budget-friendly and just as nutritious as animal sources.

-

Dairy and Alternatives: Dairy products provide calcium, vitamin D, and protein, which are important for bone health. If you're lactose intolerant or following a vegan diet, consider fortified plant-based alternatives like almond, soy, or oat milk.

-

Fats: Healthy fats, found in foods like avocados, nuts, seeds, and olive oil, are important for brain health and hormone production. While fats should be consumed in moderation, they are an essential part of a balanced diet.

A balanced diet doesn't have to be expensive. By planning your meals and choosing budget-friendly options from each food group, you can nourish your body without breaking the bank.

Key Nutrients on a Budget

When eating on a budget, it's important to focus on nutrient-dense foods—those that provide the most nutrients for the least amount of money. Here are some key nutrients to prioritize and affordable sources for each:

-

Protein: As mentioned earlier, protein is essential for a variety of bodily functions. Budget-friendly protein sources include eggs, beans, lentils, canned tuna, and peanut butter. These foods are versatile and can be used in a wide range of dishes.

-

Fiber: Fiber is important for digestive health and can help keep you feeling full, which is especially helpful when trying to stretch your food budget. Affordable high-fiber foods include oats, whole wheat bread, brown rice, beans, lentils, and fruits like apples and bananas.

-

Vitamins and Minerals: Fruits and vegetables are packed with vitamins and minerals, but they don't have to be fresh to be nutritious. Frozen and canned options are often more affordable and just as healthy. Look for items without added sugars or salt to keep them as healthy as possible.

●

Healthy Fats: While healthy fats can sometimes be pricey, there are budget-friendly options. For example, a small amount of olive oil goes a long way, and bulk purchases of nuts and seeds can be cost-effective. Peanut butter is another affordable option that provides healthy fats along with protein.

●

Calcium and Vitamin D: Dairy products and fortified plant-based alternatives are the best sources of these nutrients. Look for sales on milk, yogurt, and cheese, or consider buying in bulk to save money. Fortified cereals can also be a good source of vitamin D.

By focusing on these key nutrients and their budget-friendly sources, you can ensure that your diet is not only affordable but also rich in the essential components your body needs to thrive.

Common Misconceptions About Healthy Eating

There are several misconceptions about healthy eating, particularly when it comes to the cost. Let's address some of the most common myths:

●

Myth 1: Healthy Food is Always Expensive
Many people believe that eating healthy requires buying expensive superfoods or organic produce. However, this isn't necessarily true. While some health foods can be pricey, there are plenty of affordable options that are just as nutritious. For example, beans, lentils, frozen vegetables,

and whole grains are all inexpensive and packed with nutrients.

●

Myth 2: You Need to Shop at Specialty Stores
You don't need to shop at health food stores to eat well. Most grocery stores carry a wide range of healthy foods, often at lower prices. By sticking to the perimeter of the store, where fresh produce, dairy, and meats are located, and avoiding the processed foods in the center aisles, you can make healthier choices without paying a premium.

●

Myth 3: Healthy Eating Takes Too Much Time
Another common misconception is that preparing healthy meals is time-consuming. While it's true that some healthy recipes require more preparation, there are plenty of quick and easy options available. Batch cooking, using a slow cooker, or choosing simple recipes with few ingredients can help you eat well without spending hours in the kitchen.

●

Myth 4: You Have to Give Up Your Favorite Foods
Eating healthy doesn't mean you have to completely overhaul your diet or give up the foods you love. It's about making smarter choices and finding balance. For instance, you can enjoy your favorite pasta dish by using whole wheat pasta and adding plenty of vegetables, or satisfy your sweet tooth with homemade desserts that use natural sweeteners.

By debunking these myths and focusing on practical, budget-friendly strategies, this book aims to make healthy eating accessible for everyone. The key is to approach your diet with flexibility and creativity, using the tools and tips provided in the following chapters to create a plan that works for you.

Chapter 2: Smart Grocery Shopping Strategies

One of the most effective ways to eat healthy on a budget is to master the art of smart grocery shopping. By planning ahead, taking advantage of sales, and making informed choices at the store, you can stretch your food budget without sacrificing nutrition. This chapter will guide you through essential strategies to help you get the most value from your grocery shopping.

Planning Your Shopping List

A well-thought-out shopping list is your first line of defense against overspending and making unhealthy choices. Here's how to create a list that will help you stay on track:

- **Start with a Meal Plan**: Before you head to the store, take some time to plan your meals for the week. Consider your schedule, the ingredients you already have on hand, and any dietary goals you're working towards. Planning your meals in advance will help you avoid last-minute takeout and ensure you have everything you need to prepare healthy meals at home.

- **Organize by Category**: Divide your shopping list into categories, such as produce, dairy, grains, and proteins. This will make your shopping trip more efficient and help you avoid wandering into aisles where you might be tempted to buy items you don't need.

- **Include Staple Items**: Keep a list of staple items that you regularly use, such as olive oil, spices, and canned goods. Having these items on hand will make it easier to whip up meals without needing a special trip to the store.

-

Stick to Your List: Once your list is complete, commit to sticking to it. Avoid adding items to your cart that aren't on the list, unless you come across a great deal on something you know you'll use.

Navigating Sales and Discounts

Sales and discounts can be a great way to save money, but only if you approach them strategically. Here are some tips for making the most of sales:

- **Know the Sales Cycle**: Many grocery stores have regular sales cycles, with certain items going on sale at predictable intervals. Pay attention to these cycles and plan your shopping around them. For example, if you know chicken tends to go on sale every few weeks, plan to stock up when prices drop.

- **Use Coupons Wisely**: Coupons can be a valuable tool, but only if they're for items you actually need. Don't be tempted to buy something just because you have a coupon. Instead, look for coupons on items you already plan to buy or for brands you prefer.

- **Compare Unit Prices**: When items are on sale, it's easy to assume you're getting a good deal, but that's not always the case. Take the time to compare unit prices (the price per ounce, pound, or liter) to ensure you're getting the best value. Sometimes, a larger size may seem more expensive but actually offers a better price per unit.

- **Take Advantage of Loyalty Programs**: Many grocery stores offer loyalty programs that provide discounts, coupons, and rewards for frequent shoppers. Signing up for these programs can lead to significant savings over time.

Buying in Bulk vs. Buying Fresh

Deciding when to buy in bulk and when to buy fresh can have a big impact on your grocery budget. Here's how to make the right choice:

- **Buying in Bulk**: Bulk buying can be a great way to save money on non-perishable items like grains, beans, pasta, and spices. It's also a good option for items that you use frequently or can store for a long time, such as nuts, seeds, and cooking oils. However, avoid buying perishable items in bulk unless you're sure you can use them before they spoil.

- **Buying Fresh**: Fresh produce, dairy, and meats are best bought in smaller quantities, as they have a limited shelf life. Focus on buying seasonal produce, which is often cheaper and more flavorful than out-of-season items. If you find a good deal on fresh produce, consider freezing it for later use.

- **Warehouse Stores vs. Regular Grocery Stores**: Warehouse stores can offer significant savings on bulk items, but it's important to compare prices and ensure you have the storage space for large quantities. Sometimes, regular grocery stores offer better deals, especially when you take advantage of sales and discounts.

How to Avoid Impulse Buys

Impulse buys can quickly blow your budget and lead to unhealthy choices. Here are some strategies to help you avoid them:

- **Eat Before You Shop**: Shopping on an empty stomach can lead to impulsive purchases, especially of unhealthy snacks. Make sure to eat a meal or a healthy snack before heading to the store.

-

Stick to the Perimeter: The perimeter of the store is where you'll typically find fresh produce, meats, dairy, and other whole foods. Avoid the center aisles, where processed and packaged foods are often displayed. If you need items from these aisles, go directly to them and avoid browsing.

-

Use a Basket Instead of a Cart: If you're only picking up a few items, use a basket instead of a cart. The limited space will make it harder to add unnecessary items and keep you focused on what you really need.

-

Set a Budget and Bring Cash: Setting a budget for your shopping trip and bringing only the cash you plan to spend can help you resist the temptation to overspend. When you're out of cash, you're done shopping.

-

Avoid Eye-Level Temptations: Stores often place high-margin items at eye level to encourage impulse buys. Be aware of this tactic and focus on your list instead of what's directly in front of you.

Understanding Food Labels and Expiration Dates

Knowing how to read food labels and understand expiration dates can help you make healthier and more cost-effective choices. Here's what to look for:

-

Reading Food Labels: Food labels provide important information about the nutritional content of a product, including calories, fat, sugar, and sodium. Look for products with lower levels of added sugars and sodium, and opt for those with higher fiber and protein content. The ingredients list is also key—shorter lists with recognizable ingredients are generally better.

- **Understanding Expiration Dates**: Expiration dates can be confusing, but they're important for ensuring food safety and quality. Here are the most common types:
  - **"Sell By"**: This date tells the store how long to display the product for sale. It's not a safety date.
  - **"Best By"**: This date indicates when the product will be at its best quality. It's not an expiration date.
  - **"Use By"**: This is the last date recommended for using the product while at peak quality. For perishable items, it's best to follow this date closely.
  - **"Expires On"**: This date is for food safety, particularly on products like baby formula. Don't consume these products after the expiration date.

- **When to Buy Generic**: Many generic or store-brand products are just as nutritious as their brand-name counterparts and are often much cheaper. Compare labels and ingredients to make sure you're getting the same quality.

By mastering these smart grocery shopping strategies, you'll be well-equipped to make healthier choices that align with your budget. Remember, the goal is to plan ahead, make informed decisions, and avoid the common pitfalls that can lead to overspending. With these strategies, you'll be able to shop with confidence, knowing that you're getting the best value for your money while nourishing your body with nutritious foods.

Chapter 3: Meal Planning for Success

Meal planning is a powerful tool that can save you time, money, and stress while helping you maintain a healthy diet. By planning your meals in advance, you can avoid last-minute takeout, reduce food waste, and make the most of your grocery budget. This chapter will guide you through the process of meal planning, batch cooking, and creatively using leftovers to ensure you're eating well without overspending.

The Benefits of Meal Planning

Meal planning offers numerous benefits that can make a significant difference in both your wallet and your well-being:

- **Saves Time**: By planning your meals for the week, you eliminate the daily question of "What's for dinner?" You'll spend less time in the kitchen and more time enjoying your meals and the other activities you love.

- **Reduces Food Waste**: When you plan your meals, you buy only what you need. This reduces the likelihood of food spoiling before you have a chance to use it, which means you're not throwing money away on unused groceries.

- **Promotes Healthier Eating**: With a meal plan in place, you're less likely to reach for unhealthy convenience foods. You'll have balanced, nutritious meals ready to go, making it easier to stick to your dietary goals.

- **Saves Money**: Planning your meals allows you to take advantage of sales, buy in bulk, and avoid impulse purchases. You'll also be able to repurpose ingredients across multiple meals, getting the most value out of what you buy.

•

Reduces Stress: Knowing that your meals are planned and prepped can take a significant amount of stress out of your day. You'll have more mental space to focus on other important aspects of your life.

Creating a Weekly Meal Plan

Creating a weekly meal plan doesn't have to be complicated. Here's a step-by-step guide to get you started:

1. **Assess Your Week**: Begin by looking at your calendar. Consider your schedule, including any nights when you'll be working late, attending events, or dining out. This will help you determine how many meals you need to plan for.
2. **Choose Your Recipes**: Select recipes that fit your schedule and dietary needs. Look for meals that share common ingredients to save money and reduce waste. Consider a mix of easy-to-prepare dishes for busy nights and more involved recipes when you have more time.
3. **Make a Shopping List**: Once you've chosen your recipes, make a shopping list of all the ingredients you'll need. Be sure to check your pantry, fridge, and freezer to avoid buying duplicates.
4. **Plan for Leftovers**: Intentionally plan meals that will create leftovers, which can be used for lunches or repurposed into new dishes later in the week. This is a great way to maximize the value of your grocery purchases.
5. **Stick to Your Plan**: Once your plan is in place, commit to following it. Flexibility is important, but try to stay on track to avoid unnecessary trips to the grocery store or ordering takeout.

How to Batch Cook and Store Meals

Batch cooking is an excellent strategy for saving time and money while ensuring you have healthy meals ready to go throughout the week. Here's how to do it effectively:

- **Choose Recipes That Scale**: When batch cooking, select recipes that can be easily doubled or tripled without compromising flavor or texture. Soups, stews, casseroles, and grain-based salads are all great options for batch cooking.

- **Prep in Advance**: Dedicate a specific day or time for meal prep. Start by chopping vegetables, marinating proteins, and cooking grains in large quantities. This will make the actual cooking process faster and more efficient.

- **Use the Right Storage Containers**: Invest in quality storage containers that are microwave-safe, freezer-friendly, and leak-proof. Glass containers are a good choice as they're durable and don't retain odors. Portion out your meals into individual containers for easy grab-and-go options during the week.

- **Label and Date**: Always label and date your containers before storing them in the fridge or freezer. This will help you keep track of what needs to be eaten first and prevent food waste.

- **Freeze for Later**: If you're making a large batch of a particular dish, consider freezing half of it for later use. This is especially useful for busy weeks when you don't have time to cook. Be sure to cool foods completely before freezing to maintain their quality.

-

Reheat Safely: When reheating frozen meals, do so thoroughly to ensure they reach a safe internal temperature. Soups and stews can be reheated on the stove, while casseroles and other dishes can be reheated in the oven or microwave.

Tips for Using Leftovers Creatively

Leftovers don't have to be boring. With a little creativity, you can transform them into entirely new meals. Here are some ideas to help you make the most of what's in your fridge:

- **Reinvent Proteins**: Leftover chicken, beef, or pork can be shredded and used in tacos, sandwiches, salads, or stir-fries. Add some fresh vegetables and a different sauce or seasoning to give the dish a new flavor profile.
- **Repurpose Grains**: Cooked grains like rice, quinoa, or farro can be turned into fried rice, grain bowls, or added to soups and stews. Mix them with beans, vegetables, and a protein for a hearty, nutritious meal.
- **Soup It Up**: Leftover vegetables, meats, and grains can easily be combined into a soup or stew. Simply add broth, spices, and any other ingredients you have on hand for a comforting meal.
- **Create a New Dish**: Use leftovers as the base for a new dish. For example, leftover roasted vegetables can be blended into a sauce, added to a frittata, or mixed with eggs for a breakfast scramble. Stale bread can be turned into croutons or used in a bread pudding.
- **Make a Wrap or Sandwich**: Almost any leftover can be turned into a wrap or sandwich with the addition of a

tortilla, bread, or lettuce leaves. Add some cheese, sauce, or a fresh veggie to make it more interesting.

-

Freeze for Later: If you have leftovers that you don't feel like eating right away, consider freezing them for a future meal. This works especially well for soups, stews, and casseroles.

By incorporating these meal planning strategies into your routine, you'll find that eating healthy on a budget becomes much easier. Not only will you save time and money, but you'll also enjoy a more organized and stress-free approach to meals. Whether you're cooking for yourself or a family, these tips will help you make the most of your resources while ensuring you always have something nutritious and delicious on hand.

Chapter 4: Budget-Friendly Breakfast Ideas

Breakfast is often called the most important meal of the day, and with good reason. A nutritious breakfast can kickstart your metabolism, give you the energy to face the day, and set a healthy tone for the meals that follow. But eating a balanced breakfast doesn't have to be expensive or time-consuming. This chapter will provide you with a variety of budget-friendly breakfast ideas that are quick to prepare, packed with nutrients, and easy on your wallet.

Quick and Nutritious Breakfasts

When you're short on time in the morning, it's tempting to skip breakfast or grab something unhealthy on the go. However, with a little planning, you can enjoy a quick, nutritious breakfast that will fuel your day. Here are some ideas:

- **Greek Yogurt with Fruit and Nuts**: Greek yogurt is an affordable source of protein and probiotics. Top it with fresh or frozen fruit and a handful of nuts or seeds for added fiber and healthy fats. You can even prep individual portions the night before to save time in the morning.

- **Whole Grain Toast with Toppings**: Whole grain toast is a versatile and budget-friendly option. Top it with avocado and a sprinkle of salt, peanut butter and banana slices, or cottage cheese and a drizzle of honey for a satisfying breakfast that takes just minutes to prepare.

- **Microwave Scrambled Eggs**: If you're in a rush, you can make scrambled eggs in the microwave. Simply whisk eggs in a microwave-safe bowl, season with salt and pepper, and microwave in short intervals, stirring in between. Add some leftover veggies or cheese for extra flavor.

- **Instant Oatmeal with Add-Ins**: Instant oatmeal packets are convenient and inexpensive. To boost their nutritional value, add in fruits like apples or berries, a spoonful of nut butter, or a sprinkle of cinnamon. Look for low-sugar or plain varieties and customize them to your taste.

- **Breakfast Burritos**: Wrap scrambled eggs, beans, and a little cheese in a whole wheat tortilla for a portable breakfast. You can make a batch of these burritos ahead of time and freeze them, then just microwave one for a quick meal on busy mornings.

Overnight Oats and Smoothies

Overnight oats and smoothies are perfect for those who want a nutritious breakfast ready to go as soon as they wake up. Both options are customizable, affordable, and easy to prepare in advance.

- **Overnight Oats**: To make overnight oats, simply combine rolled oats with your choice of milk (dairy or plant-based) in a jar or container. Add in your favorite mix-ins, such as chia seeds, honey, fruit, or nuts. Let it sit in the fridge overnight, and in the morning, you'll have a delicious, ready-to-eat breakfast. Some popular flavor combinations include:

  - **Peanut Butter Banana**: Oats, milk, peanut butter, sliced banana, and a dash of cinnamon.

  - **Berry Almond**: Oats, milk, mixed berries, sliced almonds, and a drizzle of honey.

Apple Cinnamon: Oats, milk, diced apple, cinnamon, and a sprinkle of walnuts.

- **Smoothies**: Smoothies are a great way to pack a lot of nutrients into a quick meal. You can use frozen fruits and vegetables, which are often cheaper and last longer than fresh ones. To make a balanced smoothie, include a mix of fruits, vegetables, a protein source (like Greek yogurt, protein powder, or peanut butter), and a liquid (such as water, milk, or juice). Here are a few budget-friendly smoothie ideas:

  - **Green Smoothie**: Spinach, banana, frozen mango, Greek yogurt, and water.

  - **Berry Blast**: Frozen mixed berries, a handful of oats, almond milk, and a spoonful of flaxseeds.

  - **Peanut Butter Banana**: Banana, peanut butter, a scoop of protein powder, and milk.

You can prep smoothie ingredients in advance by portioning them into freezer bags. In the morning, just add the contents of a bag to your blender with your liquid of choice, and you'll have a nutritious breakfast in minutes.

Affordable Protein-Packed Options

A protein-rich breakfast helps keep you full and satisfied throughout the morning, preventing the urge to snack on less healthy options. Here are some affordable ways to incorporate more protein into your breakfast:

- **Eggs**: Eggs are one of the most cost-effective sources of high-quality protein. Whether you prefer them scrambled, boiled, poached, or made into an omelet, eggs are a versatile breakfast staple. For added nutrients and variety, mix in vegetables, herbs, or a sprinkle of cheese.

- **Cottage Cheese**: Cottage cheese is another protein-packed option that's easy on the budget. Enjoy it plain or topped with fruit, nuts, or a drizzle of honey. For a savory twist, add chopped tomatoes, cucumber, and a sprinkle of black pepper.

- **Protein Pancakes**: You can boost the protein content of your pancakes by adding ingredients like Greek yogurt, cottage cheese, or protein powder to the batter. Serve them with a side of fruit or a dollop of nut butter for a balanced meal.

- **Beans and Legumes**: Incorporating beans into your breakfast is a great way to add protein and fiber. Try making a breakfast burrito with scrambled eggs and black beans, or enjoy baked beans on whole grain toast for a hearty, budget-friendly meal.

- **Chia Pudding**: Chia seeds are packed with protein, fiber, and omega-3 fatty acids. To make chia pudding, combine chia seeds with your choice of milk and a sweetener, then let it sit in the fridge overnight. Top with fresh or dried fruit, nuts, or granola for added flavor and texture.

Creative Uses for Eggs and Oats

Eggs and oats are two of the most affordable and versatile breakfast ingredients. Here are some creative ways to use them that go beyond the basics:

- **Shakshuka**: Shakshuka is a flavorful dish of poached eggs in a spiced tomato sauce. It's easy to make and can be prepared using pantry staples like canned tomatoes, onions, and spices. Serve it with whole grain bread for a complete meal.

-

Savory Oatmeal: Oatmeal doesn't have to be sweet. Try making a savory version by cooking your oats with broth instead of water and topping them with a fried egg, sautéed vegetables, and a sprinkle of cheese or herbs.

-

Egg Muffins: Egg muffins are like mini omelets baked in a muffin tin. They're easy to customize with whatever vegetables, cheese, and meats you have on hand. Make a batch at the beginning of the week and store them in the fridge or freezer for a quick breakfast option.

-

Baked Oatmeal: Baked oatmeal is a hearty and satisfying breakfast that can be made in advance and reheated throughout the week. Combine oats with milk, eggs, fruit, and spices, then bake until golden brown. Serve warm with a drizzle of honey or maple syrup.

-

Oat Pancakes: Oat pancakes are a delicious alternative to traditional pancakes. Blend rolled oats into a flour-like consistency, then mix with eggs, milk, and a sweetener. Cook them on a griddle like regular pancakes, and top with your favorite fruits or syrup.

-

Spanish Tortilla: A Spanish tortilla is a thick, hearty omelet made with potatoes and eggs. It's simple to prepare and can be enjoyed hot or cold. Add onions, peppers, or other vegetables to make it even more nutritious.

These budget-friendly breakfast ideas show that you don't need to spend a lot of money to enjoy a nutritious start to your day. With a little creativity and planning, you can make delicious, satisfying breakfasts that will keep you energized and ready to take on whatever the day brings.

Chapter 5: Lunches that Won't Break the Bank

Lunchtime is an important opportunity to refuel your body, but it's also easy to overspend if you're buying meals on the go. Packing your own lunch not only saves money but also allows you to control the ingredients and ensure you're eating something healthy. In this chapter, we'll explore budget-friendly lunch ideas that are easy to prepare, portable, and satisfying.

Easy and Portable Lunches

When you're busy or on the move, having a lunch that's easy to transport and quick to eat is essential. Here are some ideas for portable lunches that won't break the bank:

- **Mason Jar Salads**: Mason jar salads are a convenient way to pack a fresh, healthy meal. Start with your dressing at the bottom, then layer sturdy vegetables (like cucumbers, carrots, and bell peppers), grains (like quinoa or brown rice), proteins (like chicken, beans, or tofu), and leafy greens on top. When you're ready to eat, just shake the jar and enjoy!

- **Pasta Salad**: Pasta salad is a versatile lunch option that can be made in advance and eaten cold. Use whole grain or chickpea pasta for added fiber and protein. Add in vegetables like cherry tomatoes, olives, cucumbers, and a protein like tuna, chicken, or beans. Dress with olive oil, vinegar, and your favorite herbs for a satisfying meal.

- **Rice Bowls**: Rice bowls are a great way to use up leftovers and create a balanced meal. Start with a base of brown rice or quinoa, then add vegetables, a protein, and a sauce or dressing. For example, a rice bowl with black beans, corn,

avocado, and salsa makes for a tasty, budget-friendly
lunch.

●

Wraps: Wraps are an easy-to-make, portable lunch option.
Fill a whole wheat tortilla with your choice of protein,
veggies, and a spread like hummus or yogurt-based
dressing. Some ideas include a turkey and avocado wrap, a
hummus and veggie wrap, or a chicken Caesar wrap.
Wraps can be prepared the night before for a quick grab-
and-go lunch.

●

Bento Boxes: Bento boxes are a fun and creative way to
pack a balanced lunch. Divide your meal into sections with
a variety of foods, such as sliced vegetables, a protein (like
boiled eggs, cheese, or chicken), a small portion of grains,
and a piece of fruit or nuts. Bento boxes are visually
appealing and encourage portion control.

Meal Prep for Weekday Lunches

Meal prepping your lunches for the week can save you time,
money, and stress. Here's how to get started with lunch meal prep:

●

Plan Your Menu: Begin by planning your lunches for the
week. Consider recipes that use similar ingredients to
minimize waste and save money. For example, if you're
making a quinoa salad, you can also use quinoa in a
different dish later in the week.

●

Batch Cook: Choose recipes that are easy to make in large
quantities, such as soups, stews, or casseroles. Cook a big
batch at the beginning of the week, then portion it out into
individual containers for each day. This way, you'll have a
healthy lunch ready to go without any extra effort.

●

Use Versatile Ingredients: Focus on ingredients that can be used in multiple meals, such as roasted vegetables, grilled chicken, or cooked grains. For example, roasted vegetables can be added to a salad, mixed into a grain bowl, or served as a side dish.

•

Invest in Quality Containers: Durable, leak-proof containers are essential for meal prepping. Look for containers that are microwave-safe and stackable for easy storage. Glass containers are a good option as they don't retain odors and can be used in the microwave.

•

Freeze for Later: If you have extra portions, consider freezing them for later use. This is especially useful for soups, stews, and casseroles that freeze well. Label your containers with the contents and date, so you know what you have on hand.

Budget-Friendly Salad Ideas

Salads are a nutritious and versatile lunch option, but they don't have to be expensive. Here are some budget-friendly salad ideas that are filling and full of flavor:

•

Chickpea Salad: Chickpeas are an affordable source of protein and fiber. Combine cooked chickpeas with diced cucumber, cherry tomatoes, red onion, and parsley. Dress with olive oil, lemon juice, salt, and pepper for a simple and refreshing salad.

•

Kale and Quinoa Salad: Kale is a nutrient-dense leafy green that holds up well in salads. Toss chopped kale with cooked quinoa, roasted sweet potatoes, and a handful of cranberries or nuts. Dress with a tangy vinaigrette made from olive oil, apple cider vinegar, and Dijon mustard.

-

Lentil and Veggie Salad: Lentils are another budget-friendly protein option. Cooked lentils can be combined with chopped vegetables like bell peppers, carrots, and celery, and tossed with a light dressing of olive oil, lemon juice, and herbs. This salad is hearty and can be made in advance.

-

Greek Salad: A classic Greek salad is made with cucumbers, tomatoes, red onion, olives, and feta cheese. It's a simple, yet flavorful, salad that can be made on a budget. Add a protein like grilled chicken or chickpeas to make it more filling.

-

Coleslaw Salad: Coleslaw is an inexpensive way to enjoy a crunchy salad. Use a mix of shredded cabbage, carrots, and green onions, and toss with a light dressing made from yogurt, apple cider vinegar, and a touch of honey. Add sliced almonds or sunflower seeds for extra crunch.

Healthy Sandwich and Wrap Alternatives

While sandwiches and wraps are classic lunch options, there are many ways to make them healthier and more budget-friendly. Here are some alternatives to traditional sandwiches:

-

Lettuce Wraps: Instead of using bread or tortillas, try using large lettuce leaves to wrap your fillings. Romaine or butter lettuce works well for wraps. Fill with your favorite sandwich ingredients like turkey, cheese, and veggies, or go for a more Asian-inspired filling with grilled chicken, cucumber, and hoisin sauce.

-

Stuffed Pitas: Whole wheat pitas are a great alternative to traditional bread and can be stuffed with a variety of fillings. Try a Mediterranean-inspired pita stuffed with hummus, cucumber, tomato, and feta, or a more classic option with deli turkey, avocado, and greens.

- **Veggie-Packed Quesadillas**: Quesadillas are an easy and affordable lunch option that can be made healthier by packing them with vegetables. Use whole wheat tortillas and fill with a mix of sautéed veggies, beans, and a sprinkle of cheese. Serve with salsa or Greek yogurt for dipping.

- **Open-Faced Sandwiches**: By using just one slice of bread, you can cut down on carbs and calories while still enjoying a satisfying sandwich. Top your bread with avocado, smoked salmon, cucumber, and a sprinkle of herbs for a light and delicious lunch.

- **Rice Paper Rolls**: Rice paper rolls are a fun and healthy alternative to sandwiches. Fill them with thinly sliced vegetables, protein (like shrimp, tofu, or chicken), and fresh herbs. Serve with a dipping sauce like peanut or soy sauce for extra flavor. These rolls are portable and can be made in advance.

These budget-friendly lunch ideas are designed to help you eat well without overspending. With a little creativity and planning, you can enjoy a variety of delicious, nutritious lunches that keep you energized throughout the day.

Chapter 6: Affordable Dinners the Whole Family Will Love

Dinner is often the most anticipated meal of the day, a time to unwind and enjoy a satisfying meal with family or friends. However, feeding a family can be expensive, and it's easy to fall into the trap of relying on costly convenience foods. This chapter offers a variety of budget-friendly dinner ideas that are nutritious, delicious, and sure to please everyone at the table.

One-Pot and Sheet-Pan Meals

One-pot and sheet-pan meals are lifesavers for busy weeknights. They require minimal cleanup, save time, and are easy on the budget. Here are some ideas to get you started:

- **One-Pot Pasta**: One-pot pasta is a quick and easy dinner option that can be made with pantry staples. Simply combine your pasta, vegetables (like spinach, cherry tomatoes, and onions), and protein (such as beans, chicken, or sausage) in a single pot with water or broth. As the pasta cooks, it absorbs the flavors, creating a delicious, all-in-one meal. Finish with a sprinkle of cheese or fresh herbs.

- **Sheet-Pan Chicken and Vegetables**: Sheet-pan dinners are incredibly versatile and allow you to cook everything at once. Toss chicken thighs or drumsticks with your favorite vegetables (like potatoes, carrots, and bell peppers) in olive oil, garlic, and herbs. Spread everything out on a sheet pan and roast in the oven until the chicken is golden and the vegetables are tender. This meal is perfect for busy nights and can easily be scaled up for larger families.

- **One-Pot Chili**: Chili is a hearty, protein-rich meal that can be made in one pot and feeds a crowd. Use a mix of ground

beef or turkey, beans, tomatoes, and spices to create a
flavorful dish. Serve with cornbread or over rice for a
filling and budget-friendly dinner. Leftovers can be frozen
for future meals.

-

Sheet-Pan Fajitas: Fajitas are a family favorite that can be
easily made on a sheet pan. Toss sliced bell peppers,
onions, and chicken strips with fajita seasoning and olive
oil. Spread them out on a sheet pan and roast until the
chicken is cooked through and the vegetables are tender.
Serve with warm tortillas, salsa, and guacamole for a
complete meal.

-

One-Pot Stir-Fry: Stir-fries are a great way to use up
leftover vegetables and create a quick, healthy dinner. In a
large pan or wok, cook your choice of protein (like tofu,
chicken, or shrimp) with garlic and ginger. Add a variety of
vegetables and cook until tender. Finish with a simple
sauce made from soy sauce, sesame oil, and a touch of
honey. Serve over rice or noodles.

Protein-Rich Dinners on a Budget

Getting enough protein doesn't have to be expensive. There are
plenty of budget-friendly protein options that can be used to create
satisfying dinners:

-

Beans and Legumes: Beans and legumes are among the
most affordable sources of protein. They can be used in a
variety of dishes, from soups and stews to salads and
casseroles. Try making a bean and vegetable stew, lentil
curry, or black bean tacos for a protein-rich meal that's
easy on the wallet.

-

Egg-Based Dishes: Eggs are a versatile and inexpensive protein source. Consider making a frittata, quiche, or shakshuka for dinner. These dishes are easy to customize with whatever vegetables, cheese, or herbs you have on hand.

-

Canned Tuna or Salmon: Canned fish is a budget-friendly way to add protein and omega-3 fatty acids to your diet. Use canned tuna or salmon to make patties, add to pasta dishes, or mix into a salad. Tuna casseroles and salmon cakes are also family-friendly options that won't break the bank.

-

Chicken Thighs and Drumsticks: Chicken thighs and drumsticks are often cheaper than breasts and are just as versatile. They can be roasted, grilled, or used in casseroles and soups. Try marinating them in your favorite sauce before cooking for extra flavor.

-

Tofu and Tempeh: Tofu and tempeh are plant-based proteins that are affordable and versatile. They can be stir-fried, grilled, or baked, and easily absorb the flavors of marinades and sauces. Use tofu in a stir-fry, tempeh in a grain bowl, or either in a curry for a filling and nutritious dinner.

Vegetarian and Plant-Based Options

Eating more plant-based meals is not only good for your health, but it's also good for your budget. Here are some vegetarian and plant-based dinner ideas that are both hearty and affordable:

-

Vegetable Stir-Fry: Stir-fries are a quick and easy way to enjoy a variety of vegetables in one meal. Use a mix of fresh or frozen vegetables, such as broccoli, bell peppers, carrots, and snap peas. Add tofu or tempeh for protein, and serve over brown rice or noodles with a simple stir-fry sauce.

-

Stuffed Peppers: Stuffed peppers are a great way to use up leftover grains and vegetables. Cut the tops off bell peppers and remove the seeds. Stuff them with a mixture of cooked rice or quinoa, beans, corn, and salsa. Top with a sprinkle of cheese and bake until the peppers are tender.

-

Vegetarian Chili: Vegetarian chili is a filling and nutritious dinner that's easy to make in large batches. Use a mix of beans, lentils, tomatoes, and vegetables, along with your favorite chili spices. Serve with cornbread or over a baked potato for a complete meal.

-

Pasta Primavera: Pasta Primavera is a simple and budget-friendly dish that highlights fresh vegetables. Cook your choice of pasta and toss with sautéed vegetables like zucchini, cherry tomatoes, and bell peppers. Finish with olive oil, garlic, and a sprinkle of Parmesan cheese.

-

Sweet Potato and Black Bean Tacos: Tacos don't need to include meat to be delicious. Roast diced sweet potatoes with cumin and chili powder, and serve them in tortillas with black beans, avocado, and salsa. These tacos are flavorful, filling, and easy on the budget.

Comfort Food Without the Cost

Comfort food doesn't have to be expensive or unhealthy. With a few budget-friendly tweaks, you can enjoy your favorite comfort dishes without breaking the bank:

-

Homemade Macaroni and Cheese: Macaroni and cheese is a classic comfort food that's easy to make from scratch. Use whole grain pasta and make a simple cheese sauce with milk, butter, and shredded cheese. For extra nutrition, stir in some steamed broccoli or spinach before baking.

-

Shepherd's Pie: Shepherd's pie is a hearty dish that combines ground meat with vegetables, topped with mashed potatoes. To make it more budget-friendly, use ground turkey or a mix of lentils and mushrooms in place of ground beef. The result is a comforting, filling meal that everyone will love.

-

Chicken and Rice Casserole: Chicken and rice casserole is a simple, one-dish meal that's perfect for feeding a family. Combine cooked rice with cooked chicken, vegetables, and a creamy sauce made from broth and a little bit of cheese. Bake until bubbly and golden for a comforting dinner.

-

Beef and Bean Chili: Chili is a budget-friendly comfort food that's easy to make in large batches. Use a mix of ground beef or turkey, beans, tomatoes, and spices to create a hearty dish that can be served with cornbread or over rice. Leftovers can be frozen for a quick meal later on.

-

Vegetable Pot Pie: Vegetable pot pie is a comforting dish that's easy to make with budget-friendly ingredients. Use a mix of frozen vegetables and a simple sauce made from broth and flour. Top with a homemade or store-bought pie crust, and bake until golden brown. This dish is perfect for a cozy family dinner.

These affordable dinner ideas prove that you don't have to spend a lot to enjoy a delicious, satisfying meal with your family. By using budget-friendly ingredients and simple cooking techniques, you can create a wide variety of dinners that everyone will love.

Chapter 7: Snacks and Sides on a Budget

Snacks and sides are often overlooked when planning meals on a budget, but they play an important role in maintaining a balanced diet and curbing hunger between meals. With a little creativity and smart planning, you can enjoy healthy, satisfying snacks and sides without overspending. This chapter will provide you with budget-friendly ideas for snacks and side dishes, as well as tips for making the most of your snacking habits.

Healthy Snacks to Curb Hunger

Snacking doesn't have to mean reaching for something unhealthy. With a few simple ingredients, you can create snacks that are nutritious, filling, and easy on your budget:

- **Fruit and Nut Butter**: Pairing fresh fruit with a spoonful of nut butter is a quick and satisfying snack. Apples, bananas, and celery are affordable options that go well with peanut butter or almond butter. This combination provides a good balance of natural sugars, fiber, and healthy fats.

- **Yogurt with Toppings**: Plain Greek yogurt is a high-protein snack that can be customized with a variety of toppings. Add fresh or frozen fruit, a drizzle of honey, or a sprinkle of granola for added flavor and texture. To keep costs down, buy yogurt in larger tubs rather than single-serving containers.

- **Veggies and Hummus**: Fresh vegetables like carrots, cucumbers, and bell peppers are perfect for dipping in hummus. Hummus is easy to make at home with canned chickpeas, tahini, lemon juice, garlic, and olive oil. This snack is both nutritious and satisfying.

-

Popcorn: Popcorn is a low-cost, whole-grain snack that's easy to make at home. Air-pop your popcorn and season it with a sprinkle of salt, nutritional yeast, or cinnamon for a healthy and tasty treat. Avoid pre-packaged microwave popcorn, which can be expensive and high in unhealthy fats.

-

Hard-Boiled Eggs: Hard-boiled eggs are an inexpensive, protein-rich snack that's easy to prepare in advance. They can be eaten on their own, sliced on whole-grain toast, or paired with veggies for a more substantial snack.

Affordable Homemade Snack Recipes

Making your own snacks at home can save you money and help you avoid the unhealthy additives often found in store-bought snacks. Here are some budget-friendly homemade snack recipes:

-

Energy Bites: Energy bites are a simple, no-bake snack that can be made with pantry staples. Combine rolled oats, peanut butter, honey, and add-ins like chocolate chips or dried fruit. Roll into bite-sized balls and refrigerate. These bites are great for a quick pick-me-up during the day.

-

Roasted Chickpeas: Roasted chickpeas are a crunchy, protein-packed snack that's easy to make at home. Toss canned chickpeas with olive oil and your favorite spices, then roast in the oven until crispy. Store them in an airtight container for a healthy snack on the go.

-

Homemade Granola Bars: Granola bars are a convenient snack, but store-bought versions can be pricey. Make your own by combining oats, nuts, seeds, dried fruit, and honey. Press the mixture into a baking dish and bake until golden. Once cooled, cut into bars and enjoy throughout the week.

•

Banana Bread: Banana bread is a great way to use up overripe bananas and make a delicious snack. Combine mashed bananas with whole wheat flour, eggs, a touch of honey, and baking powder. Bake until golden brown. Slice and serve as a snack or breakfast treat.

•

Veggie Chips: Homemade veggie chips are a healthier alternative to store-bought potato chips. Slice vegetables like sweet potatoes, zucchini, or kale thinly, toss with olive oil and seasonings, and bake until crispy. These chips are a nutritious and satisfying snack.

Budget-Friendly Sides for Every Meal

Side dishes are an important part of any meal, adding variety and nutrition without adding much to your grocery bill. Here are some budget-friendly side dish ideas:

•

Roasted Vegetables: Roasted vegetables are an easy and inexpensive side dish that pairs well with almost any meal. Use seasonal vegetables like carrots, potatoes, or Brussels sprouts, toss with olive oil and your favorite herbs, and roast until tender. Roasted vegetables can be made in large batches and reheated throughout the week.

•

Rice and Beans: Rice and beans are a classic, budget-friendly side dish that's full of protein and fiber. Use brown rice for added nutrients and combine with black beans, kidney beans, or chickpeas. Add a dash of cumin, garlic, and lime juice for extra flavor.

•

Coleslaw: Coleslaw is a refreshing and inexpensive side dish that can be made with just a few ingredients. Shred cabbage and carrots, then toss with a simple dressing made

from yogurt, apple cider vinegar, and a touch of honey.
Coleslaw pairs well with grilled meats or sandwiches.

*

Mashed Potatoes: Mashed potatoes are a comforting side
dish that's easy to make on a budget. Use russet or Yukon
Gold potatoes, boil until tender, and mash with a little
butter and milk. For extra flavor, add garlic or herbs like
chives or parsley.

*

Quinoa Salad: Quinoa is a versatile grain that can be used
in a variety of side dishes. Cook quinoa and toss with diced
vegetables, beans, and a simple vinaigrette. This salad can
be served warm or cold and makes a great side for grilled
meats or as a light lunch on its own.

Smart Snacking Tips

Snacking can be a healthy part of your diet if done mindfully. Here
are some tips to help you snack smarter while staying within your
budget:

*

Plan Your Snacks: Just as you plan your meals, plan your
snacks for the week. This will help you avoid impulse
purchases and ensure you have healthy options on hand.
Keep a variety of snacks available so you can choose
something that satisfies your cravings without
overspending.

*

Portion Control: It's easy to overeat when snacking,
especially with items like nuts or chips. Portion out your
snacks into individual servings to avoid eating more than
you intended. Use small containers or snack bags to make
it easier to grab a portioned snack on the go.

*

Stay Hydrated: Sometimes, what we perceive as hunger is actually thirst. Before reaching for a snack, try drinking a glass of water and waiting a few minutes. Staying hydrated can help you avoid unnecessary snacking and keep you feeling full.

-

Choose Nutrient-Dense Snacks: Focus on snacks that provide a good balance of nutrients, including protein, fiber, and healthy fats. These types of snacks will keep you fuller for longer and provide sustained energy, helping you avoid the temptation to reach for less healthy options.

-

Avoid Processed Snacks: Processed snacks are often high in sugar, unhealthy fats, and preservatives, and they can be more expensive than homemade alternatives. Whenever possible, choose whole, unprocessed foods for your snacks. Fresh fruits, vegetables, nuts, and whole grains are all great options.

With these budget-friendly snack and side ideas, you can keep hunger at bay and round out your meals without overspending. By planning ahead and making smart choices, you'll be able to enjoy a variety of healthy, satisfying snacks and sides that fit within your budget.

Chapter 8: Desserts Without the Guilt

Dessert is often the highlight of a meal, but it's easy to overindulge in sweets that are high in sugar and cost. The good news is that you can still enjoy delicious desserts without the guilt by choosing healthier, low-cost options that satisfy your sweet tooth without breaking the bank. This chapter will explore budget-friendly dessert ideas, healthy alternatives to traditional sweets, and tips for enjoying desserts in moderation.

Low-Cost, Low-Sugar Dessert Ideas

Desserts don't have to be loaded with sugar to be enjoyable. Here are some low-cost, low-sugar dessert ideas that are both satisfying and easy to make:

- **Fruit Salad**: A fresh fruit salad is a simple, naturally sweet dessert that's both nutritious and affordable. Use a mix of seasonal fruits like berries, apples, oranges, and grapes. For added flavor, toss the fruit with a squeeze of lemon juice and a sprinkle of cinnamon. You can also add a dollop of yogurt or a handful of nuts for extra texture and protein.

- **Baked Apples**: Baked apples are a warm, comforting dessert that requires just a few ingredients. Core the apples and fill the center with a mixture of oats, cinnamon, and a drizzle of honey. Bake until the apples are tender, and serve with a spoonful of Greek yogurt or a sprinkle of nuts.

- **Frozen Yogurt Bark**: Frozen yogurt bark is a refreshing and low-sugar treat that's easy to make. Spread a layer of plain Greek yogurt on a baking sheet lined with parchment paper. Top with fresh or frozen berries, nuts, and a drizzle of honey or dark chocolate. Freeze until solid, then break into pieces for a quick, guilt-free dessert.

-

Banana Ice Cream: Banana ice cream is a creamy, dairy-free dessert that's naturally sweet and budget-friendly. Simply freeze ripe bananas, then blend them in a food processor until smooth. You can add a splash of vanilla extract, cocoa powder, or peanut butter for extra flavor. Serve immediately or freeze for a firmer texture.

-

Chia Seed Pudding: Chia seed pudding is a versatile dessert that's low in sugar and high in fiber. Combine chia seeds with your choice of milk and a touch of honey or maple syrup. Let it sit in the fridge overnight to thicken. In the morning, you'll have a pudding-like dessert that can be topped with fruit, nuts, or granola.

Healthy Alternatives to Traditional Sweets

Traditional desserts can be high in sugar, unhealthy fats, and calories. By making a few simple swaps, you can create healthier versions of your favorite treats without sacrificing flavor:

- **Whole Wheat or Almond Flour**: Replace white flour with whole wheat or almond flour in your baking to add more fiber and nutrients. These flours have a slightly nutty flavor that pairs well with many desserts, such as muffins, cookies, and cakes.

- **Natural Sweeteners**: Instead of refined sugar, try using natural sweeteners like honey, maple syrup, or mashed bananas. These options are sweeter and often contain more nutrients than processed sugar. For example, you can replace sugar with mashed bananas in banana bread or use honey in homemade granola bars.

- **Greek Yogurt**: Greek yogurt is a healthier alternative to sour cream or heavy cream in desserts. Use it in place of these ingredients in recipes like cheesecakes, parfaits, or frosting. Greek yogurt is lower in fat and higher in protein, making your desserts more nutritious.

-

Dark Chocolate: Dark chocolate contains less sugar than milk chocolate and is rich in antioxidants. Use dark chocolate in place of milk chocolate or white chocolate in recipes like brownies, cookies, or chocolate bark. The rich flavor of dark chocolate means you can use less and still get a satisfying treat.

-

Avocado: Avocado can be used as a healthy fat substitute in desserts like brownies, mousse, or frosting. Its creamy texture and mild flavor make it a perfect base for chocolate desserts. Avocado is packed with healthy fats, fiber, and vitamins, making it a nutritious addition to your sweets.

Baking on a Budget: Simple Recipes

Baking at home is a great way to control the ingredients in your desserts and save money. Here are some simple, budget-friendly baking recipes to try:

-

Oatmeal Cookies: Oatmeal cookies are a classic, budget-friendly dessert that's easy to make. Combine rolled oats, whole wheat flour, a natural sweetener, and your choice of add-ins like raisins, nuts, or dark chocolate chips. These cookies are satisfying and can be enjoyed as a snack or dessert.

-

Banana Bread: Banana bread is a great way to use up overripe bananas and make a delicious dessert or breakfast treat. Mix mashed bananas with whole wheat flour, eggs, a touch of honey, and baking powder. You can also add nuts or dark chocolate chips for extra flavor. Bake until golden brown and enjoy warm or at room temperature.

●

Apple Crisp: Apple crisp is a warm, comforting dessert that's perfect for using up apples. Slice apples and toss them with a little cinnamon and honey, then top with a mixture of oats, whole wheat flour, and a small amount of butter. Bake until the topping is golden and the apples are tender. Serve with a scoop of Greek yogurt or a dollop of whipped cream.

●

Peanut Butter Cookies: Peanut butter cookies are a simple, gluten-free dessert that requires just a few ingredients. Mix peanut butter with a natural sweetener, an egg, and a pinch of baking soda. Form into balls, flatten with a fork, and bake until golden. These cookies are rich, satisfying, and easy to make.

●

Pumpkin Muffins: Pumpkin muffins are a healthy and budget-friendly dessert that can also be enjoyed for breakfast. Combine pumpkin puree with whole wheat flour, eggs, a natural sweetener, and spices like cinnamon and nutmeg. Bake until golden brown and enjoy with a cup of tea or coffee.

Tips for Moderation and Portion Control

Even healthy desserts should be enjoyed in moderation. Here are some tips for practicing portion control and avoiding overindulgence:

●

Serve Smaller Portions: Start by serving smaller portions of dessert. Use smaller plates or bowls to help control portions visually. If you're still hungry, wait a few minutes before deciding if you want more.

-

Share Desserts: Sharing desserts with family or friends is a great way to enjoy a treat without overindulging. When dining out, consider splitting a dessert with someone else. At home, cut larger desserts into smaller portions and share them.

-

Savor Each Bite: Take the time to savor each bite of your dessert. Eating slowly and mindfully can help you feel more satisfied with a smaller portion. Focus on the flavors, textures, and aromas of your dessert, and enjoy the experience.

-

Freeze Extra Portions: If you've made a large batch of dessert, consider freezing extra portions for later. This can help you avoid the temptation to eat too much at once. When you're ready for another treat, simply thaw a portion from the freezer.

-

Balance with Healthy Meals: If you know you'll be having dessert, balance it with healthy meals throughout the day. Focus on eating plenty of fruits, vegetables, whole grains, and lean proteins to keep your diet balanced and nutritious.

By incorporating these low-cost, low-sugar dessert ideas and healthy alternatives into your diet, you can enjoy sweet treats without the guilt. With a focus on moderation and portion control, you'll be able to satisfy your sweet tooth while maintaining a healthy, balanced diet.

Chapter 9: Special Dietary Needs on a Budget

Navigating special dietary needs can be challenging, especially when you're trying to stick to a budget. Whether you're gluten-free, dairy-free, vegan, or managing food allergies, it's possible to eat well without overspending. This chapter will provide tips and meal ideas for accommodating special dietary needs in a budget-friendly way.

Gluten-Free and Dairy-Free Options

Eating gluten-free or dairy-free doesn't have to be expensive. By focusing on whole foods and avoiding processed gluten-free or dairy-free products, you can maintain a healthy diet without breaking the bank.

- **Gluten-Free Grains**: Many naturally gluten-free grains are affordable and versatile. Rice, quinoa, millet, and buckwheat are all great options that can be used in a variety of dishes. Use them as a base for grain bowls, salads, or as a side dish with vegetables and proteins.

- **Dairy-Free Milk Alternatives**: Dairy-free milk alternatives, such as almond, soy, or oat milk, are widely available and often affordable. To save money, consider making your own milk alternatives at home. For example, homemade oat milk can be made by blending oats with water and straining the mixture. It's a cost-effective and easy way to enjoy dairy-free milk.

- **Gluten-Free Pasta and Bread**: While gluten-free pasta and bread can be pricey, look for store brands or buy in bulk when they're on sale. You can also make your own gluten-free bread or pasta at home using affordable ingredients like rice flour, cornstarch, and tapioca flour.

- **Dairy-Free Yogurt and Cheese**: Dairy-free yogurt and cheese can be more expensive than their dairy counterparts. To save money, look for store brands or make your own dairy-free yogurt using coconut milk or almond milk. Nutritional yeast is an affordable ingredient that can be used as a cheesy topping for pasta, popcorn, or salads.

- **Gluten-Free Baking**: Baking gluten-free at home is often more economical than buying pre-made gluten-free baked goods. Stock up on gluten-free flours like rice flour, almond flour, and coconut flour when they're on sale. Use these flours to make muffins, cookies, or pancakes that are gluten-free and budget-friendly.

Vegan and Vegetarian Budget Meals

Plant-based diets are not only healthy but can also be budget-friendly. By focusing on whole foods and making use of affordable staples like beans, lentils, and vegetables, you can create delicious vegan and vegetarian meals on a budget.

- **Beans and Legumes**: Beans and legumes are some of the most affordable sources of protein and fiber. Use them in soups, stews, salads, and grain bowls. Canned beans are convenient and often inexpensive, but dried beans are even more budget-friendly and can be cooked in large batches.

- **Tofu and Tempeh**: Tofu and tempeh are versatile plant-based proteins that are often less expensive than meat. Use tofu in stir-fries, curries, or grilled dishes, and tempeh in sandwiches, salads, or as a meat substitute in tacos. Marinate them in your favorite sauces for added flavor.

- **Seasonal Vegetables**: Buying seasonal vegetables is a great way to save money while eating a variety of nutrient-dense foods. Plan your meals around what's in season, and look for deals at farmers' markets or discount grocery stores. Vegetables like carrots, potatoes, cabbage, and leafy greens are often available year-round at affordable prices.

- **Whole Grains**: Whole grains like brown rice, quinoa, barley, and oats are filling and affordable. They can be used as the base for many vegan and vegetarian dishes. Cook grains in large batches and use them throughout the week in different meals to save time and money.

- **Meat Substitutes**: While some meat substitutes can be expensive, you can create your own using affordable ingredients like beans, lentils, mushrooms, and nuts. For example, make your own veggie burgers by combining black beans with oats, spices, and vegetables. These homemade options are often healthier and more economical than store-bought versions.

Managing Food Allergies Without Overspending

Managing food allergies can make grocery shopping more challenging, but with careful planning, it's possible to accommodate dietary restrictions without overspending.

- **Read Labels Carefully**: When managing food allergies, it's essential to read labels carefully. Look for store brands that offer allergen-free products at a lower cost than specialty brands. Many stores now have their own lines of allergen-free foods that are more affordable.

-

Cook from Scratch: Cooking from scratch allows you to control the ingredients and avoid potential allergens. It's also often more cost-effective than buying pre-packaged allergen-free foods. Focus on simple, whole foods like fruits, vegetables, grains, and proteins that you know are safe to eat.

•

Substitute Ingredients: Learn to substitute common allergens with budget-friendly alternatives. For example, use applesauce or mashed bananas as an egg substitute in baking, or replace dairy with coconut milk or oat milk. Many affordable ingredients can be used as substitutes in recipes without compromising flavor or texture.

•

Buy in Bulk: If you find allergen-free products that work for you, consider buying them in bulk to save money. Many online retailers offer bulk discounts on allergen-free flours, grains, and snacks. Just be sure to store them properly to maintain freshness.

•

Grow Your Own: If you have space, consider growing your own fruits, vegetables, or herbs. This can help you avoid potential cross-contamination from pesticides or fertilizers that may contain allergens. Plus, gardening can be a cost-effective way to access fresh produce.

Kid-Friendly Meals on a Budget

Feeding kids on a budget can be tricky, especially when trying to accommodate picky eaters or special dietary needs. Here are some tips for creating kid-friendly meals that are both nutritious and affordable:

•

Make It Fun: Presentation can make a big difference in getting kids excited about healthy meals. Use cookie cutters to create fun shapes with fruits, vegetables, or sandwiches. Arrange food in colorful patterns on the plate or create a "build-your-own" meal where kids can choose their ingredients.

-

Involve Kids in Cooking: Involving kids in the cooking process can help them feel more connected to their food and more likely to eat it. Let them help with simple tasks like washing vegetables, stirring ingredients, or setting the table. Cooking together can also be a fun and educational activity.

-

Sneak in Vegetables: If your kids are resistant to vegetables, try sneaking them into their favorite dishes. Add finely chopped spinach to pasta sauce, blend carrots into smoothies, or mix grated zucchini into muffins. This way, they'll get the nutrients they need without even realizing it.

-

Batch Cooking and Freezing: Kids often have busy schedules, so having ready-to-eat meals on hand can be a lifesaver. Batch cook kid-friendly meals like pasta dishes, casseroles, or soups, and freeze them in individual portions. This makes it easy to reheat a nutritious meal in minutes.

-

Affordable Snacks: Kids love snacks, but store-bought options can be expensive and unhealthy. Make your own snacks at home, such as popcorn, homemade granola bars, or yogurt parfaits with fruit and granola. These options are more budget-friendly and allow you to control the ingredients.

By focusing on whole foods, making smart ingredient substitutions, and involving kids in the cooking process, you can create meals that accommodate special dietary needs without overspending. With these tips and ideas, you'll be able to provide healthy, delicious meals for your family, regardless of dietary restrictions.

Chapter 10: Long-Term Strategies for Eating Healthy on a Budget

Creating and maintaining healthy eating habits on a budget is not just about saving money in the short term; it's about building a sustainable lifestyle that will benefit your health and finances in the long run. This chapter will explore strategies for building a sustainable grocery budget, the benefits of seasonal and local eating, how to grow your own food at home, and resources to help you stay on track.

Building a Sustainable Grocery Budget

A well-planned grocery budget is the foundation of eating healthy on a budget. It allows you to make the most of your money while ensuring you have access to nutritious foods. Here's how to build a sustainable grocery budget:

- **Track Your Spending**: The first step to building a grocery budget is understanding how much you're currently spending. Track your grocery expenses for a few weeks to get an accurate picture of where your money is going. Identify any areas where you might be overspending, such as impulse buys or convenience foods.

- **Set a Realistic Budget**: Based on your spending habits and financial situation, set a realistic grocery budget. Consider factors like the size of your household, dietary needs, and food prices in your area. Make sure your budget is achievable and allows for flexibility when necessary.

- **Prioritize Essentials**: When planning your grocery list, prioritize essential items like fruits, vegetables, whole grains, and proteins. Focus on nutrient-dense foods that provide the most value for your money. Avoid spending

too much on non-essential items like snacks or sugary
beverages.

-

Plan Your Meals: Meal planning is key to sticking to your
grocery budget. Plan your meals for the week based on
what's on sale and what you already have on hand. This
will help you avoid buying unnecessary items and reduce
food waste.

-

Use Cash or a Prepaid Card: One way to stick to your
budget is to use cash or a prepaid card for grocery
shopping. This limits your spending to the amount you've
allocated and prevents you from overspending. If you
prefer using a credit or debit card, make sure to track your
spending closely.

-

Adjust as Needed: Your grocery budget may need to
change over time due to changes in your income, family
size, or dietary needs. Regularly review your budget and
make adjustments as needed to ensure it remains
sustainable.

The Importance of Seasonal and Local Eating

Eating seasonally and locally not only supports your budget but
also benefits your health and the environment. Here's why it's
important and how you can incorporate it into your lifestyle:

-

Cost Savings: Seasonal produce is often less expensive
than out-of-season fruits and vegetables because it's more
abundant and requires less transportation. By focusing on
what's in season, you can enjoy fresh, nutritious foods at a
lower cost.

-

Better Flavor and Nutrition: Seasonal produce is harvested at its peak, which means it's fresher, more flavorful, and often more nutritious. Eating in season allows you to enjoy fruits and vegetables when they're at their best.

-

Support Local Farmers: Buying local produce supports local farmers and reduces the carbon footprint associated with transporting food over long distances. Many farmers' markets offer fresh, seasonal produce at competitive prices, and you can often find deals on "imperfect" fruits and vegetables that taste just as good.

-

Preserving Seasonal Produce: When certain fruits and vegetables are in season, consider buying them in bulk and preserving them for later use. You can freeze, can, or dry seasonal produce to enjoy throughout the year. This not only saves money but also allows you to enjoy your favorite fruits and vegetables year-round.

-

Seasonal Eating Guide: To help you get started, create a seasonal eating guide for your region. This will give you an idea of which fruits and vegetables are in season at different times of the year, helping you plan your meals and grocery shopping accordingly.

Growing Your Own Food at Home

Growing your own food is one of the most effective ways to eat healthy on a budget. Whether you have a large garden or just a small balcony, here's how you can start growing your own produce at home:

-

Start Small: If you're new to gardening, start with a few easy-to-grow plants like herbs, lettuce, or tomatoes. These plants require minimal space and can be grown in containers if you don't have a garden. As you gain experience, you can expand your garden to include other fruits and vegetables.

- **Choose the Right Plants**: When selecting plants, consider your climate, space, and the time you can commit to gardening. Choose plants that thrive in your local environment and are well-suited to your gardening space. If you're short on time, opt for low-maintenance plants that don't require frequent watering or care.

- **Use Cost-Effective Methods**: Gardening doesn't have to be expensive. Save money by starting plants from seeds instead of buying seedlings, using compost or natural fertilizers, and repurposing containers for planting. You can also save seeds from fruits and vegetables you buy to plant in your garden.

- **Grow Perennial Plants**: Perennial plants come back year after year, making them a cost-effective option for your garden. Consider planting perennials like berries, asparagus, or herbs that will provide a continuous harvest without the need for replanting each season.

- **Community Gardening**: If you don't have space for a garden at home, consider joining a community garden. Many communities offer shared gardening spaces where you can grow your own produce alongside other gardeners. Community gardens are also a great way to learn from experienced gardeners and share resources.

Resources and Tools for Continued Success

Maintaining healthy eating habits on a budget requires ongoing effort and access to the right resources. Here are some tools and resources to help you stay on track:

- **Meal Planning Apps**: There are several apps available that can help you plan your meals, create shopping lists, and track your grocery spending. Some popular options include Mealime, Paprika, and Yummly. These apps often include budget-friendly recipes and allow you to customize your meal plan based on your dietary needs.

- **Budgeting Tools**: Using a budgeting tool or app can help you manage your grocery budget more effectively. Apps like Mint, YNAB (You Need a Budget), or EveryDollar can track your expenses, categorize your spending, and help you stay within your budget.

- **Cookbooks and Blogs**: There are many cookbooks and blogs dedicated to budget-friendly, healthy eating. Some popular resources include *Good and Cheap* by Leanne Brown, *Budget Bytes* by Beth Moncel, and *The Frugal Girl* blog. These resources offer recipes, tips, and advice for eating well on a budget.

- **Local Resources**: Take advantage of local resources like farmers' markets, community-supported agriculture (CSA) programs, and food co-ops. These organizations often offer fresh, local produce at lower prices than grocery stores. Some communities also have food banks or discount grocery programs that provide access to affordable, nutritious food.

- **Support Groups and Forums**: Joining online support groups or forums focused on budget-friendly, healthy eating can provide motivation, ideas, and encouragement. Platforms like Reddit, Facebook, and dedicated forums offer communities where you can share tips, recipes, and success stories with others who are on the same journey.

●

Educational Workshops: Look for workshops or classes on gardening, cooking, or budgeting in your community. Many local extension offices, libraries, or community centers offer free or low-cost classes that can help you build skills and knowledge to support your healthy eating goals.

By implementing these long-term strategies, you can build a sustainable lifestyle that supports both your health and your budget. With the right tools, resources, and mindset, you can continue to eat well without overspending, making healthy eating a lasting part of your life.

Conclusion

Recap and Final Thoughts

Throughout this book, we've explored numerous strategies and ideas for eating healthy on a budget. From planning your meals and smart grocery shopping to cooking affordable dinners and accommodating special dietary needs, we've covered a wide range of topics to help you take control of your diet and finances. The key takeaway is that healthy eating doesn't have to be expensive or complicated. With a little planning, creativity, and knowledge, you can nourish your body and enjoy delicious meals without overspending.

Let's recap some of the key points:

- **Meal Planning**: Planning your meals in advance allows you to make the most of your grocery budget, reduce food waste, and ensure you have nutritious meals ready to go.

- **Smart Shopping**: By shopping with a list, taking advantage of sales and discounts, and focusing on seasonal and local produce, you can save money while still eating well.

- **Budget-Friendly Recipes**: We've shared a variety of affordable recipes for breakfast, lunch, dinner, snacks, and desserts that are both healthy and satisfying.

- **Special Dietary Needs**: Whether you're gluten-free, dairy-free, vegan, or managing food allergies, it's possible to eat well on a budget by focusing on whole foods and making smart ingredient substitutions.

-

Long-Term Strategies: Building a sustainable grocery budget, growing your own food, and using resources like meal planning apps and budgeting tools are all effective ways to maintain healthy eating habits over the long term.

Encouragement for Your Budget-Friendly Healthy Eating Journey

As you embark on your journey toward healthier, budget-friendly eating, remember that it's a process. You don't have to make all the changes at once. Start with small, manageable steps, such as planning your meals for the week or incorporating one budget-friendly recipe into your routine. Over time, these small changes will add up, leading to a healthier diet and more savings.

It's also important to be kind to yourself along the way. There will be times when life gets busy, and you might not stick to your meal plan or budget perfectly. That's okay! The goal is progress, not perfection. Learn from any setbacks and keep moving forward.

Eating well on a budget is not only achievable but also incredibly rewarding. You'll find that with the right strategies, you can enjoy a variety of delicious, nutritious meals while feeling good about your financial choices. Whether you're cooking for yourself, your family, or your friends, the skills and knowledge you've gained from this book will serve you well on your journey to better health and financial well-being.

Additional Resources and Recommended Reading

To continue your journey toward healthy, budget-friendly eating, here are some additional resources and recommended reading that you may find helpful:

- **Cookbooks**:
    -

Good and Cheap by Leanne Brown: A cookbook filled with recipes designed to be made on a tight budget without sacrificing flavor or nutrition.

○

Budget Bytes by Beth Moncel: A collection of simple, affordable recipes that prove you don't need to spend a lot to eat well.

- **Websites and Blogs**:

  ○

  Budget Bytes (www.budgetbytes.com): A popular blog that offers hundreds of budget-friendly recipes, meal prep tips, and grocery shopping advice.

  ○

  The Frugal Girl (www.thefrugalgirl.com): A blog that focuses on living well on a budget, with practical tips for saving money on groceries and cooking at home.

- **Meal Planning Apps**:

  ○

  Mealime: An app that helps you create meal plans based on your dietary preferences and budget. It also generates shopping lists to make grocery shopping easier.

  ○

  Paprika: A recipe manager and meal planning app that allows you to save recipes, plan meals, and create grocery lists.

- **Budgeting Tools**:

  ○

  Mint: A free budgeting app that tracks your spending, categorizes expenses, and helps you stay within your budget.

  ○

YNAB (You Need a Budget): A budgeting tool that helps you take control of your finances by creating a realistic budget and sticking to it.

- **Local Resources**:
    - Farmers' Markets: Visit your local farmers' market to find fresh, seasonal produce at competitive prices. Supporting local farmers also helps strengthen your community.
    - **Community Gardens**: If you're interested in growing your own food, look for community gardens in your area where you can rent a plot and start planting.

By using these resources and continuing to learn and explore new ideas, you'll be well-equipped to maintain a healthy diet on a budget. Remember, the journey to better health and financial well-being is a marathon, not a sprint. Keep making progress, one meal at a time.

Appendices

Grocery List Templates

A well-organized grocery list is essential for sticking to your budget and ensuring you have everything you need for healthy meals. Below are some templates you can use to create your own grocery lists. These templates are designed to help you categorize items and make your shopping trips more efficient.

Basic Grocery List Template

Produce:

- Apples
- Bananas
- Carrots
- Spinach
- Onions
- Potatoes

Grains:

- Brown rice
- Whole wheat pasta
- Quinoa
-

Oats

*

Bread

Proteins:

*

Chicken breasts

*

Ground turkey

*

Eggs

*

Canned beans (black beans, chickpeas)

*

Tofu

Dairy/Alternatives:

*

Milk or plant-based milk

*

Greek yogurt

*

Cheese

*

Butter

Pantry Staples:

*

Olive oil

*

Canned tomatoes

*

Tomato paste

- Broth (chicken, vegetable)
-

Spices (salt, pepper, garlic powder, cumin)

Snacks:

- Fresh fruit
- Nuts and seeds
- Popcorn kernels
-

Nut butter

Frozen:

- Frozen vegetables (broccoli, peas)
- Frozen berries
-

Frozen fish fillets

Weekly Grocery List Template

Meal Plan for the Week:

1. **Monday:**
   - Dinner: Grilled chicken with roasted vegetables
   - Side: Quinoa salad
1. **Tuesday:**
   -

Dinner: Black bean tacos with avocado

o

Side: Spanish rice

1. **Wednesday**:

   o

   Dinner: Vegetable stir-fry with tofu

   o

   Side: Brown rice

1. **Thursday**:

   o

   Dinner: Pasta primavera

   o

   Side: Garlic bread

1. **Friday**:

   o

   Dinner: Lentil soup with whole-grain bread

   o

   Side: Mixed green salad

Grocery List:

- **Produce**:

  o

  4 Bell peppers

  o

  2 Onions

  o

  1 Bunch of spinach

  o

  1 Head of garlic

  o

  3 Tomatoes

  o

  2 Avocados

- **Grains**:

o

Brown rice

o

Whole wheat pasta

o

Quinoa

o

Whole-grain bread

- **Proteins**:

    o

    Chicken breasts

    o

    Tofu

    o

    Lentils

    o

    Black beans (canned)

- **Dairy/Alternatives**:

    o

    Plant-based milk

    o

    Greek yogurt

- **Pantry Staples**:

    o

    Olive oil

    o

    Canned tomatoes

    o

    Vegetable broth

    o

    Spices (cumin, oregano, basil)

- **Snacks**:

    o

Fresh fruit (apples, bananas)

o

Nuts (almonds, walnuts)

o

Nut butter

Meal Planning Templates

Meal planning is key to eating healthy on a budget. Use these templates to organize your weekly meals, ensuring that you have a plan in place for breakfast, lunch, dinner, and snacks. This will help you avoid last-minute takeout and reduce food waste.

Basic Weekly Meal Planning Template

Day	Breakfast	Lunch	Dinner	Snacks
Monday	Overnight oats with berries	Greek salad with quinoa	Grilled chicken with roasted veggies	Apple slices with peanut butter
Tuesday	Scrambled eggs with spinach	Hummus and veggie wrap	Black bean tacos with avocado	Carrot sticks with hummus
Wednesday	Smoothie with spinach, banana	Leftover grilled chicken salad	Vegetable stir-fry with tofu	Yogurt with granola
Thursday	Whole-grain toast with avocado	Lentil soup with whole-grain bread	Pasta primavera	Mixed nuts

Friday	Greek yogurt with honey	Chickpea salad with mixed greens	Baked salmon with brown rice	Popcorn
Saturday	Oatmeal with banana	Tuna sandwich on whole wheat	Homemade pizza with veggie toppings	Fresh fruit
Sunday	Pancakes with fresh fruit	Quinoa bowl with roasted veggies	Lentil curry with basmati rice	Smoothie

Detailed Weekly Meal Planning Template

Day	Breakfast	Lunch	Dinner	Snacks	Prep Notes
Monday	Overnight oats with almond milk, berries	Greek salad with quinoa, feta, and olives	Grilled chicken, roasted sweet potatoes, spinach	Apple slices with peanut butter, nuts	Prep oats Sunday night, roast potatoes Monday
Tuesday	Scrambled eggs with spinach, whole-grain toast	Hummus and veggie wrap with bell peppers, cucumbers	Black bean tacos with avocado, salsa	Carrot sticks with hummus, yogurt	Cook extra black beans for Thursday's soup
Wednes	Green smoothie	Leftover grilled	Vegetable stir-fry with	Yogurt with	Cook extra rice for

day	(spinach, banana, almond milk)	chicken salad, whole-grain bread	tofu, brown rice	granola, fruit	Friday's dinner
Thursday	Whole-grain toast with avocado, scrambled eggs	Lentil soup with whole-grain bread	Pasta primavera (whole-wheat pasta, veggies)	Mixed nuts, fruit	Make extra pasta for Saturday's salad
Friday	Greek yogurt with honey, nuts	Chickpea salad (mixed greens, cucumbers, lemon dressing)	Baked salmon with brown rice, steamed broccoli	Popcorn, fresh berries	Marinate salmon in the morning
Saturday	Oatmeal with banana, cinnamon	Tuna sandwich on whole-wheat bread, side salad	Homemade pizza with whole-wheat crust, veggie toppings	Fresh fruit, yogurt	Prepare pizza dough in advance
Sunday	Whole-grain pancakes with fresh fruit	Quinoa bowl with roasted veggies, tahini dressing	Lentil curry with basmati rice	Smoothie (banana, spinach, almond milk)	Cook lentils and rice in the afternoon

These templates will help you organize your meals and shopping lists efficiently, ensuring that you stay within your budget while enjoying a variety of nutritious meals.